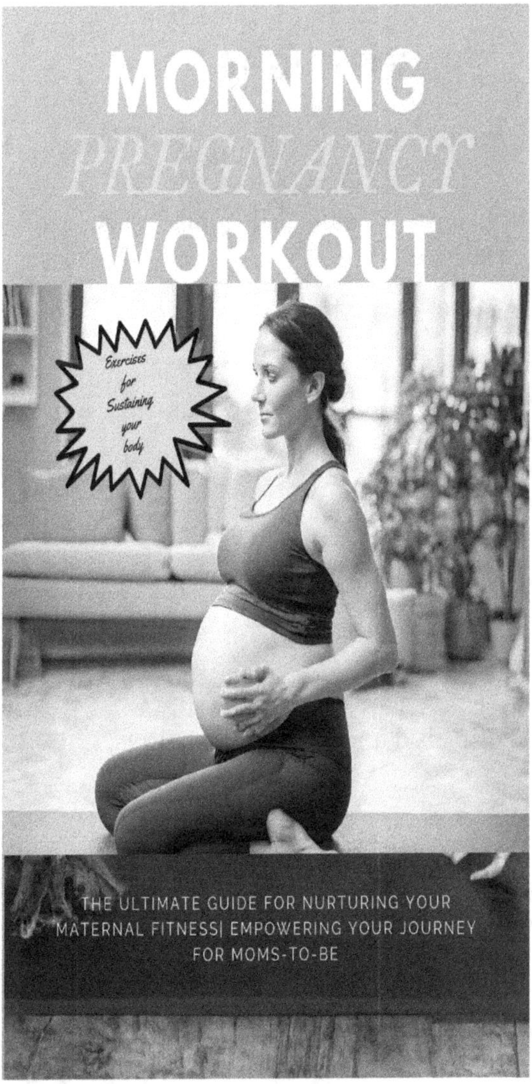

MORNING
PREGNANCY
WORKOUT
Exercises for Sustaining your body
THE ULTIMATE GUIDE FOR NURTURING YOUR MATERNAL FITNESS| EMPOWERING YOUR JOURNEY FOR MOMS-TO-BE

COPYRIGHT

©2024 Cheryl Whalen. All rights reserved.

The content and materials contained in this publication, including but not limited to text, graphics, images, audio, and video materials, are protected by copyright law and international treaties. Unauthorized reproduction, distribution, or modification of any portion of the content may result in severe civil and criminal penalties.

You may not reproduce, modify, distribute, display, perform, or transmit any of the content without prior written consent from the copyright owner.

Any unauthorized use of the content or materials may violate copyright laws, trademark laws, privacy, and publicity laws, and other applicable laws and regulations. The copyright owner reserves the right to pursue legal remedies for any unauthorized use.

TABLE OF CONTENT

CHAPTER 1

BENEFITS OF EXERCISING DURING PREGNANCY

1.1 Improved Mood

Research shows that exercising during pregnancy might improve mental and emotional health. The reference summary makes passing reference to this advantage, but more investigation into the causes of this uplift in spirits is required.

Feelings of excitement, pleasure, worry, and stress are all normal throughout pregnancy. Mood swings may be brought on by a variety of factors, including hormonal shifts, physical pains, and the excitement of expecting a child. But if you exercise regularly, you may lessen the impact of these negative feelings and develop a more optimistic outlook.

Exercise may boost mood in part because it triggers the production of feel-good endorphins. The brain releases endorphins, which have a calming and analgesic effect. Walking, swimming, or any kind of physical exercise causes your body to produce endorphins, which are feel-good chemicals that may alleviate sadness and anxiety.

Working out when pregnant also gives women a chance to prioritize their health and wellness. Expectant women sometimes put their personal needs on the back burner as they juggle the responsibilities of everyday life with those of getting ready for the birth of their baby. By setting aside specific time for exercise, women may prioritize self-care and create a good place for themselves.

Moreover, enrolling in prenatal fitness classes or joining support groups may give social connections with other pregnant women who are going through similar difficulties. This feeling of connection and shared understanding can be immensely uplifting and encouraging throughout pregnancy.

It is worth mentioning that increased mood via exercise is not confined to merely physical activities like running or yoga. Even modest stretching activities or relaxation methods like pregnant Pilates or meditation have been found to have a significant influence on mental well-being.

For example, performing deep breathing techniques during prenatal yoga sessions not only helps increase flexibility but also encourages relaxation by lowering stress levels. This combination of physical activity and mindfulness encourages pregnant women to connect with their bodies and discover a feeling of serenity despite the changes and anxieties of pregnancy.

In conclusion, exercising during pregnancy may dramatically increase mood and mental well-being. The release of endorphins, the chance for self-care, and the feeling of camaraderie all contribute to a more positive mindset. By including exercise in their daily routine, pregnant moms may better handle the emotional ups and downs that come with pregnancy.

1.2 Increased Energy Levels

One typical complaint among pregnant women is exhaustion or low energy levels. However, participating in regular exercise throughout pregnancy may assist in raising energy levels and battling symptoms of weariness.

When you exercise, your body boosts blood flow and oxygen delivery to your muscles, which helps improve general circulation. This enhanced blood flow not only helps your muscles but also offers more oxygen to your brain, resulting in greater mental alertness and higher energy.

Regular physical exercise also boosts the synthesis of mitochondria within cells. Mitochondria are crucial for turning nutrients into energy that our systems can utilize. By boosting the number of mitochondria via exercise, pregnant women may increase their body's capacity to produce energy effectively.

Furthermore, exercise helps control hormones such as cortisol, which is commonly connected with stress and exhaustion. When cortisol levels are increased for lengthy durations, it may contribute to feelings of tiredness. However, engaging in moderate-intensity workouts like brisk walking or swimming has been demonstrated to lower cortisol levels and create a more balanced hormonal state.

It is vital to remember that although exercise may enhance energy levels, it is crucial to heed to your body's signs and not overexert yourself. Pregnancy already entails extra demands on your body, so it is crucial to pick activities that are safe and suitable for each trimester.

For example,low-impact workouts like pregnant yoga or water aerobics are mild on joints while yet giving cardiovascular benefits. These sorts of exercises assist expecting moms to maintain their fitness levels without placing undue pressure on their bodies.

In addition to the physical advantages, exercise may also have a positive impact on mental energy and attention. By participating in regular physical exercise, pregnant women may have increased sleep quality, lower stress levels, and greater cognitive performance. This mental clarity and heightened alertness might contribute to overall sensations of vigor and well-being.

In conclusion, exercising during pregnancy may assist in overcoming weariness and enhance energy levels. Improved circulation, higher production of mitochondria, modulation of hormones, and improved mental energy are among the advantages that expecting moms might enjoy via regular physical activity. By including exercise in their daily routine, pregnant women might feel more invigorated and better ready to tackle the demands of pregnancy.

1.3 Reduced Discomfort

Pregnancy typically comes with many discomforts such as back pain, swollen ankles, or pelvic instability. However, exercising during pregnancy may help ease these discomforts by strengthening muscles, improving posture, and boosting flexibility.

One frequent symptom encountered by many pregnant women is back pain. As the baby develops and the center of gravity slips forward, it puts additional pressure on the lower back. However, participating in workouts that target the core muscles and encourage proper posture will help ease this ache.

Exercises like prenatal Pilates or mild strength training primarily target the deep abdominal muscles that support the spine. Strengthening these muscles helps maintain the pelvis and alleviate strain on the lower back.

Additionally, exercising good body mechanics during everyday tasks such as lifting items or getting out of bed may further avoid or lessen back discomfort.

Swollen ankles are another typical pain during pregnancy owing to fluid retention induced by hormonal changes. Regular exercise helps improve circulation throughout the body, lowering swelling in the ankles and feet.

Low-impact sports like walking or swimming stimulate blood flow from your legs back up to your heart. This activity helps avoid fluid accumulation in your lower extremities and enhances overall cardiovascular health.

Furthermore, workouts that concentrate on stretching and flexibility might help relieve pain associated with pelvic instability. As the ligaments in the pelvis relax in preparation for delivery, some women may suffer pain or discomfort in the pelvic region.

Gentle stretches and exercises that target the hip muscles may help stabilize the pelvis and ease this pain. Prenatal yoga, for example, involves positions that gently stretch and strengthen the hips, providing relief from pelvic discomfort.

In addition to bodily discomforts, exercising during pregnancy may also assist in relieving mental anguish such as worry or tension. By participating in regular physical exercise, pregnant women may relieve stress and improve calm. This may have a favorable influence on general well-being and contribute to a more pleasant pregnancy experience.

In conclusion, exercising during pregnancy may greatly reduce discomfort by strengthening muscles, improving posture, promoting circulation, and expanding flexibility. Targeted exercises for back pain, swelling ankles, and pelvic instability may bring relief from these frequent discomforts. By including exercise in their routine, pregnant moms may better manage physical discomforts and experience a more comfortable pregnancy journey.

CHAPTER 2

COMMON CONCERNS AND MISCONCEPTIONS ABOUT EXERCISING WHILE PREGNANT

2.1 Addressing Safety Concerns

Exercising during pregnancy might generate worries about safety for both expecting moms and others around them. However, it is vital to address these concerns and give comfort that exercising while pregnant may be safe and helpful when done carefully.

One major fear is the potential for damage to the infant. Many individuals fear that excessive activity or specific motions may damage the growing fetus. However, studies have shown that moderate-intensity exercise does not increase the risk of bad outcomes for the baby.

Frequent activity throughout pregnancy has been connected with a decreased risk of gestational diabetes, premature delivery, and excessive weight gain.

Another safety worry is the possible influence on the mother's cardiovascular system. Some persons fear that exercising while pregnant may strain the heart or contribute to excessive blood pressure. However, studies have indicated that women who participate in regular physical activity during pregnancy have a lower chance of developing hypertension and other cardiovascular issues.

It is vital to remember that safety issues may differ based on an individual's health state and any pre-existing medical disorders.

Expectant moms should always contact their healthcare provider before beginning or maintaining an exercise regimen during pregnancy.

Healthcare experts may give individualized advice based on an individual's particular circumstances and assist in addressing any issues connected to safety.

Additionally, pregnant women need to listen to their bodies and make adaptations as required during exercise sessions. This entails paying attention to indicators of weariness, dizziness, shortness of breath, or discomfort and adjusting intensity or taking pauses appropriately. Staying hydrated and wearing suitable clothes are also vital for preserving comfort and minimizing overheating.

By addressing these safety concerns head-on and offering evidence-based information, expecting moms may feel secure in their choice to integrate exercise into their pregnancy experience.

2.2 Debunking Myths about Exercise and Pregnancy

There are various misconceptions regarding exercise during pregnancy that might generate unwarranted worry or misunderstanding among pregnant moms. It is important to refute these stereotypes and give correct facts to assist women in making educated choices regarding their workout regimens.

One prevalent myth is exercise might trigger miscarriage. However, research has repeatedly demonstrated that moderate-intensity exercise does not raise the risk of miscarriage in healthy pregnancies. In reality, staying active throughout pregnancy may offer various advantages for both the mother and baby.

Another thing is exercise might contribute to preterm labor. While it is true that some high-impact or intense activities may pose a danger in some cases, partaking in moderate-intensity exercise has not been observed to raise the incidence of premature delivery. Frequent physical exercise throughout pregnancy has been related to a lower risk of premature birth.

There is also a myth that exercising while pregnant will affect the baby's development or growth. However, studies have repeatedly demonstrated that moderate-intensity exercise does not significantly affect fetal growth or development. On the contrary, regular physical exercise has been related to better placental function and greater fetal well-being.

It is crucial to remember that every pregnancy is unique, and individual circumstances may justify certain precautions or adaptations to exercise regimens. Consulting with a healthcare expert before beginning or maintaining an exercise program during pregnancy may assist in addressing any concerns and offer individualized instruction based on an individual's particular requirements.

By refuting these beliefs and offering factual information, pregnant moms may feel empowered to make decisions that promote their health and well-being throughout their pregnancy journey.

2.3 Reassurance and Guidance for Expectant Mothers

Pregnancy is a period filled with enthusiasm but also uncertainty for many pregnant moms. It is vital to give comfort and assistance to help people negotiate the physical changes they encounter and make informed decisions about their health.

One area where reassurance is frequently sought is body image. Pregnancy brings about considerable changes in a woman's physique, which may occasionally lead to feelings of self-consciousness or uneasiness. It is crucial to educate pregnant moms that these changes are normal and required for the growth and development of their kids. Emphasizing the beauty and strength of the pregnant body may help increase confidence and develop a good body image.

Guidance on handling discomforts often linked with pregnancy is also necessary. Many women endure back pain, pelvic girdle discomfort, or other musculoskeletal difficulties during pregnancy. Guiding on maintaining excellent posture, doing moderate stretches, and participating in exercises that target particular muscle areas may help ease these discomforts and enhance general well-being.

Furthermore, pregnant moms typically have anxieties about weight gain throughout pregnancy. It is crucial to reassure them that weight gain is a natural part of the process and is required for a healthy pregnancy. Encouraging a balanced approach to eating and activity may help regulate weight growth within established parameters while providing appropriate nutrients for both mother and baby.

Supporting mental well-being is vital throughout pregnancy.

Hormonal changes, bodily discomforts, and anxiety about birth and motherhood might lead to higher stress levels. Assisting with relaxation methods like deep breathing exercises, pregnant yoga, or meditation may help decrease stress and increase emotional well-being.

Lastly, it is vital to highlight the significance of self-care during pregnancy. Expectant moms generally emphasize the demands of their developing baby but may ignore their well-being in the process. Encouraging regular exercise, a good diet, restful sleep, and seeking assistance when required may help create a healthy balance between caring for oneself and preparing for parenthood.

By giving comfort and direction suited to the individual requirements of expectant women, we may enable them to embrace their pregnancy journey with confidence and make decisions that emphasize their health and well-being.

CHAPTER 3

GENTLE STRETCHING EXERCISES FOR PREGNANCY

3.1 Importance of Stretching during Pregnancy

Stretching is a vital component of every fitness plan, and it bears special relevance during pregnancy. As the body undergoes substantial changes to accommodate the developing baby, stretching helps to maintain flexibility, improve posture, and ease pain. It also promotes relaxation and decreases stress levels, which may have a favorable influence on both the mother and the growing baby.

One of the primary advantages of stretching during pregnancy is improved circulation. As the uterus develops, it exerts strain on blood vessels in the pelvic region, possibly leading to edema and varicose veins. Regular stretching exercises serve to enhance blood flow throughout the body, lowering these risks and enhancing overall cardiovascular health.

Stretching also serves a critical function in maintaining muscle tone and preventing muscular imbalances. As pregnancy continues, specific muscles grow tighter or weaker owing to changes in posture and weight distribution. By including targeted stretches into their routine, pregnant moms may correct these imbalances and lessen the likelihood of developing musculoskeletal disorders such as lower back discomfort or pelvic girdle pain.

Furthermore, stretching activities might assist in preparing the body for labor and delivery. By concentrating on particular muscle groups essential in birthing, such as the pelvic floor muscles and hip flexors, pregnant women may boost their strength and flexibility in these regions. This preparation may lead to an easier birth experience and assist in postpartum recovery.

It is crucial to remember that not all stretches are good for pregnant women. Certain postures or motions may place undue pressure on the abdomen or produce pain. Therefore, pregnant moms need to speak with their healthcare physician or a trained prenatal fitness specialist before commencing any stretching regimen.

3.2 Safe and Effective Stretching Techniques

When it comes to stretching during pregnancy, safety should always be a major consideration. Expectant moms should concentrate on easy stretches that should not entail jumping or jerking motions, since they might strain the muscles and increase the chance of injury. Instead, patients should choose static stretches, holding each posture for 15 to 30 seconds and breathing deeply throughout.

A wonderful beginning point for safe stretching during pregnancy is a gentle warm-up exercise. This might involve exercises such as walking or marching in place to stimulate blood flow and warm up the muscles before stretching. It is crucial to listen to the body and avoid overstretching or straining beyond comfort limits.

Some useful stretching practices for pregnant women include:

1. Cat-Cow Stretch: Start on all fours with hands exactly under shoulders and knees under hips. Inhale deeply while arching the back and elevating the head towards the ceiling (cow position). Exhale gently while rounding the back, tucking the chin towards the chest (cat stance). Repeat this pattern multiple times, concentrating on soft movements and keeping a neutral spine.

2. Hip Opener Stretch: Sit on a mat with legs outstretched in front. Bend one knee and put the foot on the opposite inner thigh. Gently bend forward, reaching towards the outstretched leg while maintaining the back straight. Hold this posture for 15 to 30 seconds, then swap sides.

3. Standing Side Stretch: Stand with feet hip-width apart and arms relaxed at your sides. Inhale deeply while extending one arm above, reaching towards the opposing side. Keep both feet planted and prevent leaning or twisting excessively. Hold for 15 to 30 seconds, then repeat on the opposite side.

4. Chest Opener Stretch: Stand tall with feet shoulder-width apart and interlace fingers behind your back. Slowly elevate your arms away from your body while pressing your shoulder blades together. Take deep breaths in this posture for 15 to 30 seconds.

Remember to constantly heed your body's suggestions during stretching exercises. If any activity causes pain or discomfort, it is crucial to stop immediately and check with a healthcare expert.

3.3 Targeted Muscle Groups for Stretching

During pregnancy, specific muscle groups are more prone to tightness or weakening owing to the changes in the body's structure and weight distribution. By concentrating on these particular muscle areas, pregnant women may decrease pain and preserve maximum performance throughout their pregnancy journey.

One of the important muscle groups that should be addressed for stretching during pregnancy is the hip flexors. These muscles, positioned at the front of the hips, might become tight and shortened due to extended sitting or increased pressure from the expanding uterus. Tight hip flexors may lead to lower back pain and pelvic discomfort. Gentle exercises such as lunges or kneeling hip flexor stretches may help lengthen these muscles and increase flexibility.

The pelvic floor muscles also play a key function during pregnancy and childbirth. These muscles support the bladder, uterus, and rectum, and they undergo major modifications during pregnancy. Strengthening and stretching exercises for the pelvic floor may help avoid disorders such as urine incontinence or pelvic organ prolapse. Kegel exercises, which include tightening and releasing the pelvic floor muscles, are highly recommended during pregnancy.

Another crucial place to work on is the lower back. As the baby grows, the center of gravity slips forward, causing increasing tension in the lower back muscles. Stretching activities that target this region may help release tension and lessen pain. Gentle activities such as sitting forward bend or child's pose might give relief to tense lower back muscles.

Additionally, stretching exercises for the chest and shoulders are beneficial during pregnancy. As the breasts develop and postural changes occur, these regions may become tight or rounded forward. Stretching techniques that open up the chest and extend the front of the shoulders may assist in improving posture and releasing stress in these regions.

It is worth emphasizing that every woman's body is unique, thus it is necessary to heed individual demands while targeting certain muscle areas for stretching. Consulting with a healthcare physician or pregnant fitness specialist may give individualized direction and verify that the stretching program is safe and effective.

In conclusion, stretching during pregnancy provides several advantages for expectant moms. It helps preserve flexibility, boosts circulation, reduces muscular imbalances, prepares the body for labor, and promotes relaxation.

By implementing safe and effective stretching exercises into their routine, pregnant women may promote their physical well-being and experience a better pregnancy journey. Targeting particular muscle groups such as the hip flexors, pelvic floor muscles, lower back, chest, and shoulders may treat frequent areas of stiffness or weakness. Remember to always emphasize safety and check with a healthcare expert before beginning any fitness regimen during pregnancy.

CHAPTER 4

CARDIO WORKOUTS FOR PREGNANCY

4.1 Benefits of Cardiovascular Exercise during Pregnancy

Cardiovascular exercise, often known as aerobic exercise, is a sort of physical activity that boosts your heart rate and breathing rate. Engaging in cardiovascular activity during pregnancy has several advantages for both the mother and the baby. While the reference summary briefly covers some of these advantages, this section will dig further into the issue, bringing additional insights and investigating topics not included in the summary.

One of the key advantages of cardiovascular activity during pregnancy is increased mood. Pregnancy might bring about hormonal changes that may lead to mood swings and elevated stress levels. Engaging in regular aerobic exercises produces endorphins, which are known as "feel-good" chemicals. These endorphins assist in improving your mood, alleviate anxiety and despair, and enhance general mental well-being.

In addition to increasing mood, cardiovascular activity also increases energy levels. Many pregnant women suffer exhaustion owing to hormonal changes and increasing demands on their bodies. However, incorporating low-impact cardio activities into your program may help battle this exhaustion by boosting blood circulation and oxygen supply throughout your body. This increased blood flow delivers a natural energy boost that may help you feel more alert and energized throughout the day.

Another notable advantage of cardiovascular activity during pregnancy is improved cardiovascular health. Regular aerobic activities build your heart muscle, expand lung capacity, and improve overall cardiovascular function. This heightened cardiovascular fitness might be especially advantageous during labor and delivery when your body needs more oxygen supply to handle the demands of childbirth.

Furthermore, participating in low-impact aerobic activities helps maintain a healthy weight increase throughout pregnancy. It is vital to emphasize that pregnancy is not a time for weight reduction; rather, it is a time to concentrate on maintaining a healthy weight for both you and your baby's well-being. Cardiovascular activity burns calories and helps prevent excessive weight gain by increasing metabolism and encouraging fat burning.

Additionally, cardiovascular activity has a key function in reducing discomfort linked with pregnancy. As your baby develops, your body undergoes substantial changes, including a rise in weight and a shift in your center of gravity. This may lead to typical discomforts such as back pain, joint pain, and edema. Low-impact aerobic activities assist in strengthening the muscles that support your spine and joints, relieving these discomforts and encouraging improved posture.

Moreover, cardiovascular activity during pregnancy has been found to reduce the incidence of gestational diabetes and preeclampsia. Gestational diabetes is a disorder defined by high blood sugar levels during pregnancy, whereas preeclampsia is a potentially hazardous illness distinguished by high blood pressure and damage to organs such as the liver or kidneys. Regular aerobic exercise helps manage blood sugar levels, enhance insulin sensitivity, and maintain healthy blood pressure levels, minimizing the chance of developing these illnesses.

Lastly, participating in cardiovascular activity throughout pregnancy may have long-term advantages for both you and your baby's health. Studies have revealed that infants born to moms who exercised frequently throughout pregnancy tend to have better birth weights and lower body fat percentages. Additionally, these newborns may have superior cognitive development later in life.

It is crucial to remember that every pregnancy is unique, and it is necessary to contact your healthcare professional before beginning or adjusting any exercise plan. They may give individualized counsel based on your unique circumstances and ensure that you participate in safe and appropriate cardiovascular activities throughout your pregnancy journey.

4.2 Low-Impact Options for Cardio Workouts

Low-impact cardio exercises are a fantastic alternative for pregnant women since they deliver all the advantages of cardiovascular exercise without putting excessive stress on the joints or risking damage. While the reference description briefly covers low-impact possibilities for cardio workouts, this part will explore numerous low-impact activities in greater depth, bringing additional insights into each option.

Walking is one of the easiest but most effective low-impact cardio exercises for pregnant women. It takes no extra equipment other than a comfortable pair of shoes and may be readily included in your daily routine. Walking not only improves your heart rate but also helps build the muscles in your legs, hips, and core. It is a safe and accessible alternative for women at all stages of pregnancy.

Swimming and water aerobics are other highly suggested low-impact cardio workouts during pregnancy. The buoyancy of the water lowers the stress on your joints while providing resistance to work against, making it a great option for cardiovascular fitness. Swimming utilizes numerous muscular groups simultaneously, including those in your arms, legs, back, and core. Additionally, being in the water helps decrease swelling and offers a refreshing feeling that may be especially useful during the later stages of pregnancy.

Cycling on a stationary bike or riding a recumbent bike is another low-impact alternative for cardio activities during pregnancy. These exercises provide cardiovascular advantages without placing pressure on your joints or risking falls. Stationary bikes enable you to tailor the intensity of your exercise by adjusting resistance levels, making it perfect for ladies with varied fitness levels. Recumbent bikes give extra support to your lower back and reduce strain on your pelvic region.

Low-impact aerobic dance courses or prenatal dance workouts are also popular alternatives for pregnant women wishing to participate in cardiac exercise while having fun. These programs often feature mild motions that increase cardiovascular fitness while emphasizing maintaining proper alignment and avoiding high-impact leaps or twists that might strain the body.

Elliptical trainers are another fantastic alternative for low-impact cardio workouts during pregnancy. These devices replicate walking or running movements without putting undue stress on your joints. They create a smooth gliding action that stimulates both your upper and lower body muscles while reducing impact forces.

Prenatal yoga or Pilates programs may also be adapted to incorporate low-impact cardiovascular workouts. While these activities generally concentrate on flexibility, strength, and relaxation, including fluid sequences or adding features such as standing poses or modest leaps may boost your heart rate and give cardiovascular benefits.

It is vital to remember that whatever the low-impact cardio exercise you pick, it is necessary to listen to your body and change the intensity as required. Pay attention to any discomfort or pain and alter your exercise appropriately. Additionally, always warm up before beginning any exercise regimen and cool down afterward to reduce muscular tightness and enhance flexibility.

4.3 Customizing Cardio Workouts to Fit Individual Fitness Levels

Customizing aerobic activities during pregnancy is vital to ensure that they are safe, effective, and suited for your unique fitness level. While the reference summary briefly covers adaptations for various phases of pregnancy and fitness levels, this section will investigate customization in more depth, bringing fresh insights into adapting cardio routines individually for each individual.

Firstly, it is crucial to evaluate your pre-pregnancy fitness level while designing your aerobic routines. If you were already physically active before becoming pregnant, you may be able to continue with similar exercises at a slightly lowered intensity. However, if you were not routinely active before pregnancy or have any underlying health concerns, it is advisable to start with low-impact workouts and gradually increase the intensity as your body adjusts.

Secondly, it is vital to take into consideration the stage of pregnancy you are in while tailoring your cardio routines. As your pregnancy advances, various alterations may be required owing to changes in balance, joint laxity, or comfort levels. For example, during the first trimester when exhaustion and morning sickness may be more frequent, concentrating on shorter-length workouts or implementing rest intervals between activities might assist in managing these symptoms.

During the second trimester when many women feel increased energy levels and less nausea, they may be able to participate in longer-duration exercises with greater intensity levels. However, it is still crucial to minimize overheating by keeping hydrated and exercising in a well-ventilated environment.

In the third trimester, as your baby develops and your center of gravity moves, it is essential to concentrate on activities that preserve stability and decrease the danger of falls or injury. This may entail decreasing the intensity or effect of specific exercises, such as substituting high-impact leaps with low-impact alternatives or altering the range of motion in particular activities.

Additionally, it is vital to listen to your body and make modifications based on how you feel throughout each training session. Pregnancy hormones may decrease joint stability and flexibility, therefore it is vital to avoid overstretching or pushing yourself too much. If you suffer any discomfort, dizziness, shortness of breath, or vaginal bleeding while exercising, it is crucial to stop immediately and talk with your healthcare physician.

Furthermore, designing cardio exercises should also take into account any unique medical issues or concerns that may occur during pregnancy. For example, if you have been diagnosed with gestational diabetes or preeclampsia, your healthcare physician may prescribe particular changes to manage these illnesses while still participating in safe cardiovascular activity.

Lastly, obtaining expert coaching from a licensed pregnant fitness instructor or speaking with your healthcare practitioner may give helpful insights into personalizing cardio programs depending on your unique requirements. These specialists can evaluate your fitness level, monitor your development during pregnancy, and give specific suggestions for safe and effective cardiac workouts.

In conclusion, tailoring cardio exercises during pregnancy is vital for guaranteeing safety and efficacy. Taking into consideration pre-pregnancy fitness levels, stage of pregnancy, individual comfort levels, and any specific medical issues helps pregnant women modify their workouts accordingly. By doing so, pregnant moms may enjoy the numerous benefits of cardiovascular exercise while reducing risks and maximizing overall well-being during their pregnancy journey.

CHAPTER 5

MODIFICATIONS FOR DIFFERENT STAGES OF PREGNANCY AND FITNESS LEVELS

5.1 Adapting Exercises for the First Trimester

During the first trimester of pregnancy, many women suffer exhaustion, nausea, and changes in their body that might impair their workout regimen. It is vital to listen to your body and make adaptations as required to achieve a safe and pleasant exercise.

One significant factor during the first trimester is the increased chance of miscarriage. While exercise is normally safe at this period, it is crucial to avoid high-impact activities or exercises that impose undue tension on the abdominal muscles. Instead, concentrate on low-impact workouts like walking, swimming, or pregnant yoga.

Another alteration to consider during the first trimester is lowering the intensity level of your exercises. Many women discover that they have less energy during this period owing to hormonal changes and morning sickness. It is crucial to heed your body's demands and not push yourself too hard. If you were previously engaged in high-intensity activities, you may need to drop down and concentrate on more moderate exercises.

Additionally, it is vital to pay attention to any warning indications or pain during activity. If you develop dizziness, shortness of breath, or pain while working out, it is crucial to stop immediately and talk with your healthcare professional. These symptoms might be an indication that you are overexerting yourself or that there may be an underlying problem.

It might also be good to seek instruction from a trained prenatal exercise instructor who can make specific changes depending on your individual requirements and fitness level. They can assist you in navigating the changes in your body and ensure that you are participating in workouts that are safe and helpful for both you and your baby.

Remember that every pregnancy is different, so what works for one woman may not work for another. It is crucial to listen to your body's indications and make modifications appropriately. As usual, contact your healthcare physician before beginning any new exercise regimen during pregnancy.

5.2 Modifying Workouts for the Second Trimester

The second trimester of pregnancy is commonly referred to as the "golden period" since many women have greater energy levels and a decrease in morning sickness. This is a fantastic time to concentrate on maintaining your fitness level and preparing your body for the physical demands of labor and delivery.

One essential alteration to consider during the second trimester is avoiding workouts that entail resting flat on your back. As your uterus expands, it may place strain on a large vein called the vena cava, which can impede blood flow to both you and the baby. Instead, choose workouts that keep you in an upright or inclined posture, such as standing or utilizing a stability ball.

Another worry during the second trimester is the relaxing of ligaments and joints owing to hormonal changes. This may increase the risk of injury, especially in high-impact activities or workouts that include abrupt movements or twisting motions. It is vital to find workouts that are low-impact and concentrate on stability and balance.

Additionally, as your belly develops, it may become more tough to maintain good form and alignment during some workouts. It is crucial to pay attention to your posture and utilize your core muscles to support your increasing tummy. Consider integrating activities that target the pelvic floor muscles, like Kegels or squats, which may aid with pelvic stability and prepare you for birth.

It is also vital to remain hydrated throughout exercises and take breaks as required. Pregnancy increases blood volume, which means you may need more water than normal to be adequately hydrated. Listen to your body's indications for thirst and take pauses when required to relax and recuperate.

Lastly, don't forget about the significance of mental well-being at this period. Pregnancy may bring up a multitude of emotions, so it is vital to choose hobbies that help you relax and decrease stress. Prenatal yoga or meditation may be fantastic alternatives for fostering calm and connecting with your body and baby.

5.3 Adjustments for Third Trimester and Postpartum Recovery

The third trimester of pregnancy brings about considerable changes in your body as you prepare for the birth of your baby. It is crucial to make further changes to your workout regimen during this period to guarantee safety and comfort.

One crucial adjustment during the third trimester is concentrating on exercises that encourage healthy fetal posture. This includes participating in activities that assist the baby to be in an optimum position for delivery, such as walking, swimming, or prenatal Pilates. These exercises may assist in strengthening the pelvic floor muscles and support the appropriate alignment of the baby's head.

As your belly continues to develop, it may become more tough to maintain balance and stability during certain workouts. Consider using props or support, such as a chair or wall, to aid with balance. You can also adjust workouts by completing them sitting or utilizing a stability ball for extra support.

It is vital to heed your body's indications and avoid any workouts that produce discomfort or agony. As you conclude your pregnancy, you may need to further lower the intensity level of your exercises and concentrate on gentle motions that encourage relaxation and prepare your body for labor.

After giving birth, it is vital to give yourself time to heal before resuming exercise. The postpartum period is a time of healing and adjustment, both physically and mentally. It is advisable to wait until you have obtained approval from your healthcare professional before commencing any workout regimen.

When you do start exercising again, begin lightly and gradually build intensity over time. Your body has gone through enormous changes throughout pregnancy and delivery, so it is crucial to be gentle with yourself while you restore strength and endurance.

Postpartum recovery exercises should concentrate on strengthening core strength, especially the deep abdominal muscles known as the transverse abdominis. moderate activities such as pelvic tilts, moderate abdominal contractions, and Kegels may assist in strengthening these muscles and facilitate healing.

In conclusion, modifying workouts for each stage of pregnancy is vital to providing a safe and successful fitness regimen. From making modifications during the first trimester to concentrating on ideal fetal posture in the third trimester, it is crucial to listen to your body's instincts and make changes as required. Additionally, postpartum recovery activities should be approached with delicacy and care, giving your body time to heal before progressively increasing intensity. By prioritizing your well-being and getting help from healthcare experts or trained prenatal fitness instructors, you may maintain a healthy and active lifestyle throughout your pregnancy experience.

CHAPTER 6

NUTRITION DURING PREGNANCY

6.1 Essential Nutrients for Mother and Baby's Health

Proper diet is vital throughout pregnancy to promote the health and development of both the mother and the baby. While it is well-known that certain nutrients are important, such as folic acid and iron, other lesser-known nutrients play a key part in maintaining a successful pregnancy.

One such vitamin is omega-3 fatty acids, notably DHA (docosahexaenoic acid). DHA is vital for the development of the baby's brain and eyes. It may be found in fatty fish like salmon, sardines, and trout. If you don't eat fish or have dietary limitations, you may opt for DHA supplements manufactured from algae.

Another vital vitamin is choline. Choline serves a key part in prenatal brain development and helps avoid neural tube abnormalities. Good sources of choline include eggs, lean meats, legumes, and cruciferous vegetables like broccoli.

Vitamin D is particularly vital during pregnancy since it assists in calcium absorption, which is required for the formation of the baby's bones and teeth. Sun exposure is one method to receive vitamin D naturally, but it may also be available in fortified dairy products or via supplementation if recommended by your healthcare physician.

Furthermore, appropriate consumption of calcium is necessary for both the mother's bone health and the baby's skeletal growth. Dairy products including milk, cheese, and yogurt are good providers of calcium. If you are lactose intolerant or follow a vegan diet, you may choose for fortified plant-based milk substitutes or check with a healthcare expert about calcium supplementation.

It's crucial to remember that although these nutrients are vital during pregnancy, they should be received via a balanced diet rather than relying only on supplements. A diversified diet that includes fruits, vegetables, whole grains, lean meats, and healthy fats will deliver most of these essential elements.

6.2 Maintaining a Balanced Diet with Morning Sickness or Food Aversions

Morning sickness and food aversions are frequent symptoms throughout pregnancy, sometimes making it tough to maintain a balanced diet.

However, some ways may assist in maintaining sufficient nutrition even when confronted with these problems.

Firstly, it's crucial to listen to your body and consume what you can handle. If particular meals produce nausea or aversions, try to discover alternatives that give equivalent nutrition. For example, if you can't handle meat, try plant-based protein alternatives like beans, lentils, or tofu.

Eating modest, regular meals throughout the day may also help manage morning sickness. Having something light and readily digested, such as crackers or toast, before getting out of bed in the morning may alleviate nausea. It's also beneficial to have snacks on hand for when hunger hits but bigger meals are tough to stomach.

Experimenting with new cooking techniques and tastes might make meals more appetizing during this period. Some ladies find that cold or room-temperature foods are easier to handle than hot ones. Adding herbs and spices to foods may also improve the taste and make them more appetizing.

If you're battling with severe morning sickness that impacts your ability to eat and drink enough, it's crucial to seek medical help. Your healthcare practitioner may offer anti-nausea drugs or other measures to guarantee appropriate nourishment for both you and your baby.

6.3 Practical Tips for Healthy Eating During Pregnancy

Maintaining a balanced diet throughout pregnancy is vital for the well-being of both the mother and the baby. Here are some practical recommendations to help you make healthier choices during your pregnancy journey:

1. Plan your meals: Take some time each week to plan your meals and snacks. This can assist in ensuring that you have a choice of nutritious alternatives easily accessible and avoid dependency on harmful convenience foods.

2. incorporate a range of fruits and veggies: Aim to incorporate a rainbow of fruits and vegetables in your diet. Different colors represent different nutrients, so by ingesting a variety, you can guarantee you're receiving a broad range of vitamins, minerals, and antioxidants.

3. Choose whole grains: Opt for whole-grain bread, pasta, rice, and cereals instead of processed grains. Whole grains are richer in fiber and give more sustained energy throughout the day.

4. Prioritize lean proteins: Include lean sources of protein such as chicken, fish, beans, lentils, tofu, and eggs in your meals. Protein is necessary for the growth and development of the newborn.

5. Stay hydrated: Drink lots of water throughout the day to stay hydrated. Aim for at least eight glasses (64 ounces) each day or more if you are physically active or live in a hot region.

6. Limit processed foods and added sugars: Processed foods frequently include high amounts of salt, harmful fats, and added sugars. Opt for whole foods wherever feasible to ensure you're receiving the most nutrients from your meals.

7. Practice proper food handling: During pregnancy, it's crucial to be mindful of food safety to avoid foodborne infections that may

affect both you and your baby. Avoid raw or undercooked meats, unpasteurized dairy products, and some kinds of seafood known to be rich in mercury.

8. Take prenatal vitamins as recommended: Prenatal supplements are designed to address any nutritional deficiencies in your diet during pregnancy. Consult with your healthcare practitioner about which supplements are suitable for you depending on your particular requirements.

Remember that every pregnancy is unique, so it's crucial to contact your healthcare practitioner or a registered dietitian who specializes in prenatal nutrition for specialized counsel suited to your particular requirements and circumstances.

In conclusion, maintaining optimal nutrition throughout pregnancy is vital for the health and development of both the mother and the baby.

Essential nutrients including omega-3 fatty acids, choline, vitamin D, and calcium play critical roles in sustaining embryonic growth and development. Despite morning sickness or food aversions, it is easy to keep a balanced diet by listening to your body, eating small frequent meals, and experimenting with different flavors and cooking techniques. By following practical tips for healthy eating during pregnancy, such as meal planning, including a variety of fruits and vegetables, choosing whole grains and lean proteins, staying hydrated, limiting processed foods and added sugars, practicing safe food handling, and taking prenatal supplements as recommended, expectant mothers can ensure they are providing their bodies with the necessary nutrients for a healthy pregnancy journey.

CHAPTER 7

POSTURE AND BODY MECHANICS DURING DAILY ACTIVITIES

7.1 Importance of Good Posture during Pregnancy

During pregnancy, keeping excellent posture is vital for the general well-being of both the mother and the baby. Good posture helps to alleviate common discomforts linked with pregnancy, such as back pain, pelvic instability, and poor circulation. It also encourages appropriate fetal positioning and minimizes the likelihood of problems during labor and delivery.

One of the key advantages of excellent posture during pregnancy is the reduction of back discomfort. As the baby develops, the center of gravity slips forward, placing additional pressure on the lower back. By keeping adequate alignment of the spine, pregnant women may distribute this weight more evenly and reduce strain on their back muscles.

Additionally, excellent posture helps to avoid pelvic instability, a disease characterized by discomfort in the pelvic area owing to misalignment or excessive movement of the pelvic joints. By preserving a neutral pelvis and engaging core muscles, pregnant women may stabilize their pelvis and prevent pain.

Proper posture also plays a role in maximizing fetal placement. When a pregnant woman maintains an upright posture with her pelvis in a neutral position, it provides more room for the baby to progress into an ideal position for delivery. This may assist in supporting a smoother labor phase and lower the probability of interventions such as cesarean sections.

To maintain proper posture throughout pregnancy, it is crucial to be attentive to body alignment whether sitting, standing, walking, or even sleeping. Sitting on an ergonomic chair with sufficient lumbar support may assist in maintaining a neutral spine posture. When standing or walking, transferring weight equally between both feet and avoiding excessive swayback or leaning forward will encourage better alignment.

It is also vital to exercise core muscles during everyday tasks to promote appropriate posture. Strengthening workouts targeting abdominal muscles may help support the spine and pelvis. Practicing yoga or Pilates under expert direction may be effective in increasing posture awareness and strengthening core muscles.

7.2 Maintaining Proper Posture when Sitting, Standing, Walking, and Lifting Objects

Maintaining appropriate posture is not confined to certain tasks but should be done throughout the day. Whether sitting, standing, walking, or lifting objects, proper posture is vital for reducing pain and increasing general well-being.

When sitting, it is crucial to find a chair that offers enough support for the lower back. Sitting on a cushion or utilizing a lumbar roll may assist in retaining the natural curvature of the spine. Avoiding crossing legs and keeping feet level on the floor may also help to improve posture.

While standing, distributing weight equally between both feet and avoiding locking knees or slouching forward is vital. Engaging core muscles and imagining a string pulling you up from the top of your head will help align the spine appropriately.

During walking, keeping an upright posture with relaxed shoulders and swinging arms naturally will encourage proper alignment. It is necessary to take frequent rests while walking for long durations to minimize weariness and pressure on muscles.

Lifting items during pregnancy takes additional care to safeguard both the mother and the baby. When lifting, it is recommended to bend at the knees rather than at the waist to prevent placing undue pressure on the back. Engaging core muscles when lifting might give extra assistance. If an item is excessively heavy or strangely formed, requesting help or utilizing adequate lifting equipment is suggested.

7.3 Preventing Common Discomforts with Correct Body Mechanics

Correct body mechanics are vital for reducing typical discomforts linked with pregnancy. By exercising good body mechanics during daily tasks, pregnant women may reduce strain on their bodies and decrease pain.

One typical symptom during pregnancy is swelling in the hands and feet owing to impaired circulation. To prevent this, it is vital to avoid lengthy periods of standing or sitting without moving. Taking frequent pauses to stretch or move about will assist in increasing blood flow and minimize edema.

Another typical sensation is round ligament pain, which is produced by stretching and straining of the ligaments that support the uterus. To prevent this, pregnant women should avoid rapid movements or fast changes in direction. It is crucial to move gently and methodically, enabling the body to acclimate and minimize strain on the ligaments.

Proper body mechanics may also assist in decreasing pelvic discomfort or pressure.

Avoiding activities that involve extensive twisting or bending at the waist might reduce strain on the pelvis. Using good lifting methods and engaging core muscles while doing regular duties may give extra support to the pelvis.

Furthermore, optimal body mechanics may help avoid urinary incontinence, a prevalent condition during pregnancy. By exercising proper posture and using pelvic floor muscles, pregnant women may strengthen their pelvic floor and improve bladder control.

Incorporating workouts, especially targeting core muscles and pelvic floor into regular routines will further optimize body mechanics and prevent discomforts. Prenatal yoga or Pilates programs offered by professional teachers may provide information on safe and efficient activities for maintaining healthy body mechanics throughout pregnancy.

In conclusion, keeping excellent posture throughout pregnancy is vital for overall well-being. It helps ease typical discomforts like as back pain and pelvic instability, promotes proper fetal placement, and minimizes the chance of problems during labor and delivery. Proper posture should be practiced when sitting, standing, walking, and lifting items to prevent discomfort and ensure a successful pregnancy journey. By incorporating correct body mechanics into everyday tasks, pregnant women may decrease pressure on their bodies and have a more pleasant pregnancy experience.

CHAPTER 8

ROUTINES FOR CORE

Strength and Stability

8.1 Strengthening the Core Muscles during Pregnancy

During pregnancy, it is vital to maintain strong core muscles to support the developing belly, improve posture, and avoid frequent discomforts such as back pain. Strengthening the core muscles might also assist in a smoother labor and delivery procedure. While many women may be reluctant to participate in core workouts during pregnancy owing to worries about safety, research has shown that with correct adaptations and coaching, it is not only safe but also helpful.

One effective approach to strengthening the core muscles during pregnancy is through pelvic floor exercises, often known as Kegels. These workouts target the deep abdominal muscles and pelvic floor muscles, which play a key role in maintaining the uterus and bladder. Performing Kegels consistently may help avoid urinary incontinence and facilitate speedier postpartum recovery.

Another safe and efficient exercise for strengthening the core during pregnancy is modified planks. Traditional planks are not recommended during pregnancy because of the additional strain they impose on the abdominal muscles. However, customized planks may give comparable advantages without sacrificing safety. To execute a modified plank, start by kneeling on all fours with your hands squarely under your shoulders. Engage your core muscles and push your knees off the ground while maintaining your back straight. Hold this pose for a few seconds before releasing it.

It is crucial to remember that every woman's body is different, and what works for one may not work for another. It is vital to listen to your body and speak with a healthcare practitioner or prenatal fitness specialist before beginning any new workout plan during pregnancy.

To further strengthen core strength during pregnancy, incorporating exercises that target the oblique muscles might be useful. Side planks or standing side bends are wonderful choices for exercising these muscles safely. Side planks may be done by laying on your side with one forearm on the ground and your feet placed on top of each other. Lift your hips off the ground, forming a straight line from your head to your feet. Hold this position for a few seconds before swapping sides.

In addition to these activities, prenatal yoga and Pilates programs may also be useful in strengthening the core muscles during pregnancy. These classes frequently concentrate on gentle exercises that stimulate the deep abdominal muscles while developing flexibility and relaxation. Attending specialized prenatal fitness classes ensures that workouts are tailored correctly for each stage of pregnancy, offering a safe and friendly atmosphere.

Real-world examples of women who have included core- core-strengthening activities during pregnancy may give inspiration and motivation. Sarah, a mother of two, discovered that routinely performing Kegels helped her retain bladder control throughout her pregnancies and recover quicker after giving birth. She noted better posture and lower back pain compared to her previous pregnancy when she did not participate in core workouts.

8.2 Safe Exercises to Improve Core Strength

Improving core strength is vital not just during pregnancy but also for general health and well-being. A strong core helps maintain the spine, improves balance, and boosts athletic performance. However, it is vital to pick safe workouts that do not place undue pressure on the abdominal muscles or endanger the safety of the infant.

One safe exercise to build core strength is pelvic tilts. This exercise targets the deep abdominal muscles while reducing tension in the lower back. To execute pelvic tilts, lay on your back with your legs bent and feet flat on the floor. Slowly tilt your pelvis forward by forcing your lower back into the floor, utilizing your abdominal muscles. Hold this posture for a few seconds before releasing.

Another safe workout option is sitting leg raises. This exercise stimulates both the core muscles and hip flexors without placing strain on the abdomen or pelvic floor. Sit in a sturdy chair with your back straight and feet flat on the floor. Slowly elevate one leg off the ground, maintaining it straight and parallel to the floor. Hold for a few seconds before lowering it back down. Repeat with the opposite leg.

Engaging in workouts that develop total body strength may also indirectly improve core strength. For example, squats are a safe and effective workout that utilizes numerous muscular groups, including the core. To do a squat, stand with your feet shoulder-width apart and toes slightly turned out. Slowly lower your body as if sitting back into a chair while maintaining your chest elevated and core engaged. Return to the beginning posture by pushing through your heels.

It is vital to remember that good form and technique are crucial when completing any workout to prevent injury or strain. If you are unsure about how to execute an activity properly or have any concerns, check with a trained fitness expert or healthcare practitioner.

Case studies may give significant insights into the advantages of safe exercises for developing core strength during pregnancy. Emily, a first-time mother, added seated leg lifts into her regular regimen during her second trimester. She observed greater stability and balance during her pregnancy, which enabled her to keep a busy lifestyle without pain or fear of falling.

8.3 Enhancing Stability and Balance for a Healthy Pregnancy

Maintaining stability and balance throughout pregnancy is critical for preventing falls and accidents, particularly while the body experiences significant changes in weight distribution. Engaging in activities that strengthen stability and balance not only minimizes the chance of accidents but also improves general coordination and confidence.

One helpful exercise for increasing stability during pregnancy is single-leg standing. This exercise helps develop the muscles essential for maintaining balance while reducing stress on the joints. Stand near a wall or hard surface for support if required. Lift one foot off the ground while balancing on the other leg. Hold this posture for as long as comfortable before switching legs.

Another useful activity is heel-to-toe walking, often known as tandem walking. This exercise tests balance by demanding exact foot placement and coordination. Start by standing with your feet together. Take a step forward, putting the heel of one foot precisely in front of the toes of the other foot. Continue walking in a straight line, keeping this heel-to-toe pattern.

Incorporating yoga or taichi into your fitness program may also significantly enhance stability and balance during pregnancy. These techniques concentrate on slow, controlled motions that stimulate the core muscles while promoting relaxation and attention. Attending prenatal yoga or taichi classes guarantees that movements are tailored correctly for pregnancy and offers a friendly atmosphere.

Real-world examples may highlight the advantages of increasing stability and balance during pregnancy. Jessica, a mother of three, discovered that practicing single-leg stands helped her maintain stability and avoid falls as her tummy became bigger with her pregnancies. She noted greater coordination and confidence in her movements, enabling her to continue engaging in activities she liked without fear of damage.

In conclusion, strengthening the core muscles during pregnancy is vital for supporting the developing belly, improving posture, and preventing discomforts such as back pain. Safe activities such as pelvic floor exercises, modified planks, side planks, and pregnant yoga or Pilates programs may successfully develop the core muscles while supporting varied phases of pregnancy. Improving core strength with safe activities like pelvic tilts, seated leg lifts, and squats is essential not just during pregnancy but also for general health. Enhancing stability and balance through activities like single-leg stands, heel-to-toe walking, yoga, or taichi minimizes the chance of falls and injuries while enhancing coordination and confidence. By adding these workouts into their regimens with correct adaptations and coaching from healthcare experts or fitness specialists, expecting moms may experience a healthy and satisfying pregnancy journey while prioritizing their well-being and that of their baby.

CHAPTER 9

EXERCISES FOR PELVIC FLOOR HEALTH

9.1 Understanding the Importance of Pelvic Floor Muscles

The pelvic floor muscles are a set of muscles positioned at the base of the pelvis that serves a key function in supporting the organs in the pelvic region, including the bladder, uterus, and rectum. These muscles work like a hammock, giving support to these organs and helping to preserve continence.

One of the primary tasks of the pelvic floor muscles is to manage urinary and fecal continence. When these muscles are weak or malfunctioning, it may lead to difficulties such as urine incontinence or fecal incontinence. This may have a substantial influence on a person's quality of life, causing embarrassment, discomfort, and even social isolation.

In addition to its role in incontinence, healthy pelvic floor muscles are also crucial for sexual function. These muscles contribute to promoting sexual pleasure by boosting blood flow to the vaginal region and giving support during intercourse. Weak or tight pelvic floor muscles may lead to difficulty with arousal, orgasm, or discomfort during sex.

Pregnancy and delivery may impose tremendous pressure on the pelvic floor muscles. The weight of the developing baby and hormonal changes during pregnancy might weaken these muscles over time. Additionally, vaginal delivery may cause straining or tearing of the pelvic floor muscles, further affecting their strength and function.

Both men and women must recognize the significance of maintaining good pelvic floor health throughout their lives. Regular exercise targeting these muscles may help prevent or treat disorders such as urine incontinence, fecal incontinence, and sexual dysfunction.

9.2 Strengthening and Relaxation Techniques for the Pelvic Floor

Strengthening exercises for the pelvic floor are vital for maintaining its health and function. One often advised exercise is called a Kegels. Kegels include tightening and releasing the pelvic floor muscles repeatedly over time to enhance their strength and endurance.

To execute Kegels, start by identifying the pelvic floor muscles. One approach to achieve this is by thinking that you are attempting to halt the flow of urine midstream. The muscles you activate to achieve this are called your pelvic floor muscles. Once you have recognized these muscles, contract them for a few seconds, then release and rest for a few seconds. Repeat this cycle several times, progressively increasing the length of the contractions as your muscles get stronger.

It is vital to remember that relaxing methods are just as critical as strengthening activities for maintaining excellent pelvic floor health. Overly tight or strained pelvic floor muscles may lead to difficulties such as discomfort during intercourse or trouble with bowel movements. Therefore, adding relaxing methods to your regimen is crucial.

One effective calming method is deep breathing. By taking slow, deep breaths and actively relaxing the pelvic floor muscles with each exhale, you may assist in relieving tension and promote relaxation in this region. Another approach is progressive muscle relaxation, where you progressively tension and then relax several muscular groups in the body, including the pelvic floor.

Incorporating both strengthening and relaxation strategies into your pelvic floor workout regimen will assist in maintaining a healthy balance in these muscles and avoid difficulties associated with either weakness or tightness.

9.3 Promoting Optimal Pelvic Floor Health during Pregnancy

Pregnancy brings about considerable changes in a woman's body, including hormonal shifts, weight growth, and increased strain on the pelvic floor muscles. Pregnant moms need to emphasize their pelvic floor health throughout pregnancy to reduce possible issues both during pregnancy and after delivery.

One key part of achieving optimum pelvic floor health during pregnancy is keeping proper posture. As the baby develops, it may exert pressure on the lower back and pelvis if appropriate alignment is not maintained. This might lead to discomfort or even agony in certain places. By exercising excellent posture when sitting, standing, walking, and lifting items, pregnant women can reduce the tension on their pelvic floor muscles and lessen the chance of developing disorders such as back discomfort or pelvic instability.

Regular exercise throughout pregnancy is also vital for ensuring optimal pelvic floor health. Low-impact workouts including walking, swimming, or prenatal yoga may help strengthen the pelvic floor muscles and improve overall muscle tone. These exercises should be undertaken under the guidance of a healthcare practitioner to ensure they are safe and suitable for each individual's particular requirements.

In addition to exercising, keeping a balanced diet and controlling weight gain during pregnancy may also contribute to good pelvic floor health.

Excessive weight gain may place extra strain on the pelvic floor muscles, possibly leading to weakening or dysfunction. By keeping a balanced diet and participating in regular physical exercise, expecting moms may promote their overall health and decrease the pressure on their pelvic floor.

Lastly, pregnant women must listen to their bodies and seek expert counsel when required. Bear in mind that every woman's anatomy is different, and what works for one may not work for another. If any questions or issues occur about pelvic floor health during pregnancy, it is crucial to check with a healthcare physician who specializes in prenatal care. They can give specialized advice and prescribe particular workouts or treatments suited to each individual's requirements.

In conclusion, knowing the significance of pelvic floor muscles, incorporating strengthening and relaxation methods into your routine, and encouraging optimum pelvic floor health throughout pregnancy are all critical parts of sustaining overall well-being. By emphasizing these regions, people may avoid or ease difficulties connected to weak or dysfunctional pelvic floor muscles and live a better lifestyle during pregnancy and beyond.

CHAPTER 10

WORKOUTS TO SUPPORT LABOR AND DELIVERY PREPARATION

10.1 Preparing the Body for Labor and Delivery

Preparing the body for labor and delivery is a key element of pregnancy that frequently goes unnoticed. While many pregnant moms concentrate on the physical changes occurring to their bodies, it is as crucial to prepare psychologically and physically for the difficult process of birthing. In this part, we will look further into the numerous methods by which you may prepare your body for labor and delivery.

One crucial component of preparing the body for labor is strengthening the pelvic floor muscles. The pelvic floor muscles serve a key function in supporting the weight of the developing baby, as well as assisting with bladder control and maintaining proper posture. Strong pelvic floor muscles may also help in pushing during birth and avoid issues such as urine incontinence postpartum.

Exercises such as Kegels are particularly useful in strengthening the pelvic floor muscles. Kegels include tightening and releasing the muscles that control urine flow. To execute Kegels, merely squeeze these muscles for a few seconds, then release. Repeat this exercise numerous times throughout the day, progressively increasing the length of each contraction.

Another key part of preparing for labor is developing overall cardiovascular fitness. Labor may be physically demanding, requiring endurance and energy. Engaging in low-impact cardio workouts such as swimming or brisk walking may assist in enhancing cardiovascular health while limiting stress on joints.

Additionally, including activities that target particular muscle areas involved in birthing might be useful. Squats are an effective workout to improve both leg muscles and pelvic floor muscles simultaneously. By practicing squats frequently throughout pregnancy, you may develop strength in your lower body, which can be helpful during labor when you need to maintain particular postures or push successfully.

It's crucial to recognize that preparing your body for labor isn't only about physical health; it also includes mental preparation. Childbirth education classes or prenatal yoga may give essential insights into the labor process and teach relaxation methods that can help manage pain and reduce anxiety during labor. These sessions generally incorporate breathing exercises, visualization methods, and mindfulness practices that may be immensely useful during birthing.

In summary, preparing the body for labor and delivery entails a comprehensive strategy that incorporates both physical and mental components.

Strengthening the pelvic floor muscles, enhancing cardiovascular fitness, practicing particular exercises targeting birthing muscles, and enrolling in childbirth education courses or pregnant yoga are all vital components of this preparation. By taking the time to prepare your body in these ways, you may boost your chances of having a gentler labor experience.

10.2 Exercises to Promote Flexibility and Mobility

Maintaining flexibility and mobility throughout pregnancy is vital for general comfort and well-being. As your body undergoes considerable changes to accommodate the developing baby, it's crucial to participate in activities that promote flexibility and mobility. In this part, we will examine numerous exercises especially developed to promote flexibility and mobility during pregnancy.

One activity that is especially useful in developing flexibility is prenatal yoga. Prenatal yoga incorporates mild stretching with deep breathing techniques to increase flexibility while also delivering relaxing benefits.

Yoga positions such as cat-cow stretch, child's pose, and sitting forward bend may assist in reducing typical discomforts such as back pain or tight hips.

Another activity that focuses on flexibility is prenatal Pilates. Pilates focuses on strengthening the core muscles while also increasing flexibility via regulated movements. Exercises such as pelvic tilts or hip circles may assist in preserving mobility in the pelvis region while strengthening the abdominal muscles.

Stretching exercises especially targeting tight regions such as the lower back or hips may also be incredibly effective. For example, a sitting figure-four stretch may help release tension in the hips by crossing one foot over the opposing knee and gently pushing down on the lifted knee.

In addition to these specific exercises, including regular full-body stretching routines in your fitness program will assist in maintaining overall flexibility. Stretching techniques such as shoulder rolls, neck stretches, and gentle twists may help reduce muscular tension and enhance the range of motion.

It's vital to remember that flexibility exercises should always be performed with care and within a comfortable range of motion. Pregnancy hormones may make joints looser, raising the risk of injury if stretching is done excessively or forcibly. Listen to your body's indications and avoid any motions that create discomfort or suffering.

Incorporating frequent activity throughout the day is also vital for preserving flexibility and mobility. Avoid lengthy periods of sitting or standing in one posture, since this may lead to stiffness and muscle imbalances. Take pauses to walk around, stretch, or execute basic exercises such as ankle circles or shoulder shrugs.

In conclusion, encouraging flexibility and mobility throughout pregnancy is essential for general comfort and well-being. Engaging in activities such as prenatal yoga, pregnant Pilates, targeted stretches, and full-body stretching regimens may help preserve flexibility while easing typical discomforts associated with pregnancy. Remember to heed to your body's indications and avoid overstretching or violent motions that may cause damage.

10.3 Strengthening Techniques for Labor and Delivery

Strengthening practices particularly adapted for labor and delivery may considerably boost your capacity to deal with the physical demands of childbirth. In this part, we will study numerous strengthening strategies that concentrate on important muscle groups involved in labor.

One key place to improve is the core muscles. Strong core muscles give stability during work postures such as squatting or kneeling.

Exercises such as planks or modified push-ups may effectively target the core muscles while simultaneously exercising other muscle groups like the arms and shoulders.

Additionally, strengthening the gluteal muscles is vital for maintaining appropriate posture throughout pregnancy and supporting the pelvis during birth. Bridges are a terrific exercise for targeting the glutes while also engaging the hamstrings and lower back muscles. To do a bridge, lay on your back with your knees bent and feet flat on the floor. Lift your hips off the ground, clenching your glutes, and hold for a few seconds before lowering back down.

Strengthening the upper body is also useful for labor and delivery. During labor, you may need to support your weight or grip onto something for stabilization. Exercises such as bicep curls or shoulder presses utilizing light weights or resistance bands may help increase strength in the arms and shoulders.

In addition to these specific exercises, including functional movements in your fitness program will further boost overall strength for labor and delivery. Functional motions replicate common tasks and engage many muscle groups concurrently. For example, carrying groceries or lifting a laundry basket may be considered functional movements that develop the arms, shoulders, and core muscles.

It's vital to remember that although strengthening exercises are useful for labor preparation, it's equally crucial to prevent overexertion or heavy weightlifting throughout pregnancy. Always speak with your healthcare physician before beginning any new fitness regimen and heed to your body's limitations.

In conclusion, including strengthening strategies in your fitness program will considerably boost your capacity to deal with the physical demands of labor and delivery. Targeting major muscular areas such as the core, glutes, and upper body via workouts like planks, bridges, or functional motions may offer the required strength needed during labor.

Remember to emphasize safety by talking with your healthcare physician and listening to your body's instincts throughout the procedure.

CHAPTER 11

LISTENING TO YOUR BODY AND ADAPTING WORKOUTS AS NEEDED

11.1 Tuning in to Your Body's Signals during Pregnancy

During pregnancy, pregnant moms need to tune in to their body's signals and listen to what it needs. This entails paying attention to any discomfort, pain, or changes that may happen during activity. While keeping active is typically helpful for both the mother and baby, it is important to alter exercises as required and emphasize safety.

One crucial component of tuning in to your body's signals throughout pregnancy is understanding the difference between typical pregnancy discomforts and warning symptoms that suggest a need to limit or cease activity. It is usual for pregnant women to suffer slight pains, exhaustion, or shortness of breath after physical exercise. However, if these symptoms grow severe or are accompanied by dizziness, vaginal bleeding, chest discomfort, or contractions, it is crucial to seek medical attention immediately.

Another crucial cue from your body is weariness. Pregnancy may be physically taxing, and it is typical for energy levels to fluctuate throughout the day. If you feel overly fatigued or drained before or during an exercise, it may be an indication that you need rest. Pushing yourself too hard while weary may raise the chance of injury and put unneeded stress on your body.

Additionally, paying attention to your heart rate and breathing patterns can provide vital insights into how your body is reacting to exercise. As a general rule, strive for moderate-intensity exercise where you can still carry on a conversation without feeling winded. If you find yourself struggling to breathe or experiencing a high heart rate even with mild exertion, it may be an indicator that you need to reduce or alter your workout intensity.

Furthermore, listening to your joints and muscles may assist in avoiding injuries and pain during pregnancy activities. The hormone relaxin secreted during pregnancy loosens ligaments and joints in preparation for delivery. While this is required for the birthing process, it also raises the risk of joint instability and damage. If you experience any pain, stiffness, or instability in your joints, it is crucial to reduce workouts that place an undue load on them and opt for low-impact alternatives.

Real-world examples may assist in explaining the necessity of tuning in to your body's cues throughout pregnancy. Let's examine the situation of Sarah, a pregnant lady who regularly attends a prenatal yoga session. During one session, she felt a strong discomfort in her lower back while trying a particular posture. Instead of pushing through the pain, Sarah immediately informs her teacher and changes her position to lessen the agony. By listening to her body's signals and modifying the activity, Sarah avoids potential harm and continues to enjoy the benefits of yoga throughout her pregnancy.

In conclusion, listening to your body's cues throughout pregnancy is crucial for maintaining a safe and productive fitness regimen. By paying attention to pain, exhaustion, heart rate, breathing patterns, and joint/muscle sensations, pregnant moms may alter their exercises as required and prioritize their well-being.

11.2 Recognizing When to Modify or Stop Exercise

Recognizing when to adjust or cease activity is a critical ability for expectant women throughout pregnancy. While being active is generally encouraged at this period, there are specific cases when changes or full cessation of exercise may be essential for the safety of both mother and infant.

One crucial aspect in determining whether to adjust or stop exercise is understanding the idea of effort levels. It is crucial not to push yourself beyond your limitations during pregnancy since it might lead to overexertion and severe injury. Monitoring your perceived exertion level using tools such as the Borg

Rating of Perceived Exertion (RPE) scale may help you gauge how hard you are working during physical exercise. If you find yourself routinely ranking your effort level over 14 on a scale of 6-20 (where 6 indicates no exertion and 20 represents maximum exertion), it may be a sign that you need to adapt or lessen the intensity of your exercises.

Another issue to consider is the influence of exercise on your body temperature. Pregnancy boosts your core body temperature, and engaging in strenuous or extended activity might further enhance it. This may affect the growing fetus. It is vital to minimize overheating by exercising in a well-ventilated setting, wearing breathable clothes, and keeping hydrated. If you have symptoms such as dizziness, nausea, excessive perspiration, or an increased heart rate that does not return to normal after rest, it may be important to moderate or halt activity to prevent overheating.

Furthermore, some medical disorders or issues during pregnancy may demand changes or full avoidance of activity.

Conditions like as preeclampsia, placenta previa, premature delivery, gestational diabetes, and certain heart or lung problems may demand specific restrictions on physical activity. It is vital to contact your healthcare professional if you have any underlying medical disorders or concerns regarding exercising during pregnancy.

Real-world examples may assist in conveying the necessity of recognizing when to reduce or cease activity during pregnancy. Let's examine the situation of Emily, who has been consistently attending a prenatal aerobics class throughout her pregnancy. During one session, she begins experiencing contractions that do not stop even after resting. Recognizing this as a warning indication, Emily immediately stops exercising and notifies her healthcare physician. After investigation, it was decided that Emily was at risk for preterm labor and needed to avoid intense activity for the duration of her pregnancy. By identifying when to cease activity and seeking professional help quickly, Emily guarantees the safety of herself and her baby.

In conclusion, understanding when to alter or cease activity is vital for maintaining a safe and healthy pregnancy. By understanding effort levels, monitoring body temperature, evaluating underlying medical conditions/complications, and listening to warning indications from your body like as contractions or prolonged discomfort, pregnant moms may make informed decisions regarding their exercise regimen.

11.3 Seeking Professional Guidance when Necessary

Seeking expert supervision throughout pregnancy is vital for maintaining the safety and efficiency of your fitness plan. While many pregnant women may safely participate in moderate-intensity exercise, there are individual characteristics and medical concerns that may need tailored guidance from healthcare practitioners or fitness specialists.

One key part of getting expert supervision is obtaining clearance from your healthcare practitioner before beginning or maintaining an exercise regimen during pregnancy. Your healthcare professional will assess your general health, any pre-existing medical issues, and any dangers linked with physical exercise. They may give specific recommendations customized to your circumstances and assist you in navigating any worries or ambiguities about exercise during pregnancy.

Additionally, speaking with a skilled prenatal fitness professional or certified personal trainer who specializes in pregnant exercise may provide valuable insights and assistance. These specialists have the knowledge and skills to build safe and successful fitness programs that target the unique demands of pregnant women. They can help you adapt workouts, guarantee good form and technique, and give continuing support throughout your pregnancy experience.

Furthermore, obtaining expert counsel becomes even more crucial if you have any underlying medical concerns or difficulties during pregnancy. Conditions such as high blood pressure, gestational diabetes, placenta previa, or a history of premature labor may necessitate additional precautions or adaptations to your workout program. Healthcare physicians and specialist fitness experts may work together to build an appropriate strategy that takes into account these unique factors.

Real-world examples may assist in demonstrating the need to seek professional counsel throughout pregnancy. Let's examine the instance of Jessica, who has been diagnosed with gestational diabetes. She wants to continue exercising but is concerned about the sort and intensity of activities that would be safe for her condition. Jessica sees both her healthcare practitioner and a certified pregnant fitness professional who collaborate to build an activity regimen that helps regulate her blood sugar levels while assuring the well-being of herself and her baby. By obtaining expert help, Jessica acquires the confidence and knowledge to exercise properly throughout her pregnancy.

In conclusion, getting expert counsel during pregnancy is essential for tailored recommendations, risk assessment, and assuring the safety and efficacy of your workout plan. Healthcare specialists and specialized fitness professionals may give vital insights, address unique concerns or medical issues, and assist you in negotiating the physical changes of pregnancy while keeping active and healthy.

CHAPTER 12

POSTPARTUM RECOVERY AND BEYOND

12.1 Importance of Postpartum Recovery

Postpartum recovery is a key period in a woman's journey after delivering birth. It is a period when the body experiences tremendous physical and emotional changes as it recovers after the childbirth process. While many new moms may be eager to go back into their pre-pregnancy habits, it is crucial to prioritize postpartum recovery for maximum well-being.

One of the key reasons why postpartum recovery is crucial is because it helps the body to repair correctly. Pregnancy and delivery put immense pressure on a woman's body, impacting different systems such as the musculoskeletal, hormonal, and cardiovascular systems. Taking the time to relax and recuperate helps these systems to return to their pre-pregnancy level gradually.

Moreover, postpartum healing plays a critical role in avoiding long-term issues. Conditions like as diastasis recti (separation of abdominal muscles), pelvic floor dysfunction, and postpartum depression may emerge if proper healing is not emphasized. By allowing the body to recuperate entirely, women may lower their chance of acquiring these issues and increase general well-being.

It is crucial to recognize that postpartum recovery goes beyond just physical healing; it also covers mental well-being. The journey into parenthood may be daunting, with emotions of weariness, worry, and even despair being normal experiences for many new moms. By concentrating on postpartum recovery, women may nurture their mental health by obtaining help from loved ones or specialists who specialize in postnatal care.

To achieve good postpartum healing, new moms need to listen to their bodies and allow themselves permission to relax. This may involve changing expectations and accepting aid from others during this period. By embracing the significance of postpartum recovery and taking active measures toward self-care, women may set themselves up for a healthy future as they navigate the pleasures and difficulties of parenting.

12.2 Exercises for Healing and Strengthening the Body After Birth

Exercises for mending and strengthening the body after birth are vital for aiding postpartum recovery. These activities not only assist in physical recovery but also help new moms restore strength, improve posture, and boost general well-being. Here, we will cover several essential activities that may be added to a postpartum workout plan.

One vital activity for postpartum rehabilitation is pelvic floor exercises, popularly known as Kegels. The pelvic floor muscles incur tremendous strain during pregnancy and delivery, resulting in weaker muscles and associated complications such as urine incontinence. By routinely exercising pelvic floor exercises, women may strengthen these muscles, enhance bladder control, and promote speedier recovery.

Another useful workout is modest abdominal engagement or core activation exercises. These exercises concentrate on reconnecting with the deep abdominal muscles that may have been strained or weakened during pregnancy. By progressively activating these muscles via controlled movements such as pelvic tilts or moderate abdominal compressions, new moms may support their lower back, improve posture, and promote abdominal muscle healing.

In addition to particular muscle-focused exercises, low-impact cardiovascular activities such as walking or swimming may be integrated into a postpartum fitness plan. These exercises assist in enhancing circulation, raising energy levels, and supporting general cardiovascular health without putting unnecessary load on the body.

It is vital to remember that every woman's postpartum experience is unique, and it is necessary to check with a healthcare practitioner before beginning any fitness regimen. They may give tailored instruction based on individual requirements and verify that workouts are safe and suitable for each stage of postpartum recovery.

Furthermore, it is crucial to approach postpartum exercise with tolerance and love towards oneself. The body has experienced considerable changes throughout pregnancy and delivery, therefore it is typical for development to take time. By concentrating on incremental development rather than quick outcomes, new mothers can build a sustainable workout regimen that helps their postpartum recovery journey.

12.3 Nurturing Your Physical and Mental Well-being as a New Mother

Nurturing physical and emotional well-being is vital for new moms as they navigate the pleasures and difficulties of parenting. The postpartum time may be physically taxing, emotionally upsetting, and mentally tiring. Therefore, it is crucial to prioritize self-care and make conscious efforts to nourish both physical and mental well-being.

One part of cultivating physical well-being is maintaining sufficient nourishment. During the postpartum period, the body needs appropriate nutrition to support healing, nursing (if relevant), and general energy levels. New moms must concentrate on having a balanced diet that includes nutrient-dense foods such as fruits, vegetables, lean meats, whole grains, and healthy fats. Additionally, keeping hydrated is vital for sustaining excellent physical health.

In addition to diet, obtaining adequate rest is crucial for physical well-being. Sleep loss is prevalent among new moms owing to the duties of caring for a baby. However, prioritizing sleep whenever feasible can significantly affect general well-being. This may mean taking brief sleep throughout the day or asking the aid of loved ones to split nighttime responsibilities.

Mental well-being plays an equally vital part in cultivating overall wellness as a new mother. It is typical for women to feel a variety of emotions at this period, including excitement, worry, grief, or even guilt.

Seeking emotional support from loved ones or attending support groups specifically geared toward new moms may give a secure area to share experiences and receive assistance.

Practicing self-compassion and having reasonable expectations are also crucial components of maintaining mental well-being. New mothers must recognize that they are trying their best in a whole new job. Taking pauses when required, participating in activities that provide pleasure or relaxation (such as reading or practicing mindfulness), and seeking professional treatment if necessary are all helpful tactics for cultivating mental well-being.

Furthermore, maintaining social relationships is vital for new moms. The postpartum period may often seem solitary, but reaching out to friends, relatives, or other new moms can give a feeling of community and support. Whether it is via in-person events, online forums, or virtual support groups, interacting with people who understand the struggles of parenting may be immensely useful.

In conclusion, nurturing physical and emotional well-being as a new mother is crucial for overall health and happiness. By emphasizing healthy nutrition, restful sleep, emotional support, self-compassion, and social connections, women may traverse the postpartum period with more comfort and resilience. Remembering that self-care is not selfish but rather vital for becoming the greatest version of oneself as a mother is crucial. By adopting these practices and making them a priority, new moms may flourish physically and psychologically during this changing period in their lives.

"MORNING PREGNANCY WORKOUT" is a thorough handbook for expectant moms who wish to maintain a healthy and active lifestyle throughout their pregnancy. The book includes a variety of information, advice, and exercises particularly intended to assist pregnant women remain active and motivated throughout the early hours.

The book starts by addressing the advantages of exercising during pregnancy, including better mood, greater energy levels, and less pain. It covers common worries and misunderstandings regarding exercising while pregnant, giving comfort and direction to expecting moms.

Each chapter gives a range of workout activities appropriate for all fitness levels. From easy stretching exercises to low-impact aerobic routines, the book gives step-by-step directions complemented by vivid graphics.

Modifications are offered for each workout to suit various stages of pregnancy and individual fitness levels.

In addition to training programs, the book also offers valuable information on nutrition during pregnancy. Readers will learn about critical nutrients required for both mother and baby's health, as well as practical recommendations for maintaining a balanced diet while managing morning sickness or food aversions.

The necessity of appropriate posture and body mechanics throughout daily activities is underlined in the book. It includes advice on keeping proper posture when sitting, standing, walking, and lifting items – all crucial aspects of minimizing typical pregnancy-related discomforts such as back pain or pelvic instability.

Written in an approachable format, "MORNING PREGNANCY WORKOUT" seeks to equip pregnant moms with the knowledge and skills to make informed choices about their health throughout pregnancy. It encourages women to listen to their bodies, change their routines as required, and seek expert help when necessary.

Overall, "MORNING PREGNANCY WORKOUT" is a fantastic resource that helps pregnant moms negotiate the physical changes of pregnancy while keeping active and healthy. With its evidence-based approach and useful guidance, this book is a necessary companion for any woman wishing to prioritize her well-being and experience a healthy and satisfying pregnancy journey.